The Essent...

Curing GERD and Heartburn

The cure for GERD, based on the role of angle of His
and posture in development of the disease

By D.S. Spade, Ph.D.

© D. S. Spade, 2018
Published March 28st 2018
ISBN: 9781980688457

Finally, the cure for GERD

This book is a must have for everyone that suffer from Gastroesophageal Reflux Disease

Based on entirely new understanding of the cause of GERD

It contains a new exercise based approach that eradicate GERD

It is effective even for the worse cases of GERD

Eliminate the need of antacids and other GERD medicine

Save thousands from cutting antacids and skipping visits to emergency rooms and hospitals

The book is also a guide that contains all you need to know about GERD, including the conventional treatment options

Includes new tips and tricks that can help people with GERD, many of which cannot be found anywhere else

Leonardo da Vinci and GERD

The proportions of the human body according to Vitruvius, or simply the Vitruvian man is a drawing by Leonardo da Vinci made around 1490.

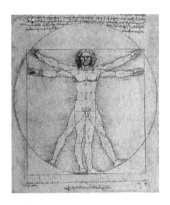

The drawing depicts the ideal proportions of the human body. As you will see in this book, GERD is a disease caused by departure from the ideal human proportions and can be cured by restoration of the anatomical and the physiological harmony of the body.

TABLE OF CONTENTS

Introduction

This book contains everything you need to know about Gastroesophageal Reflux Disease or GERD and how to overcome it. It is a must have for everyone that suffer from this disease.

The biggest asset of the book is the inclusion of a new highly effective exercise program against GERD. This program was developed in the last seven years and it is based on a new understanding of the role of the posture and the diaphragm in the development of GERD. Performing the described in this book exercises eliminates even the worst cases of the disease.

We recommend this book, especially for people that have severe form of GERD as they will be its greatest beneficiary by saving countless visits to emergencies rooms and hospitals. The book can also help people that have milder form of GERD, because the exercise program prevents the progression of the disease towards its more severe form. The exercise program also eliminates the need of antacids and other GERD medicine and can save the reader thousands in unnecessary expenses. The described exercises treat the cause GERD, in contrast to the antacid drugs such as Prilosec, Nexium and Gaviscon that treat the symptoms of the disease. This is why people can eliminate GERD by exercising, but they will never succeed in doing so only by taking the available antacid drugs.

Nevertheless, the antacids can be helpful for reducing the symptoms of GERD and especially for diagnosing the disease. This is why we have included a special chapter that contains detailed information about Prilosec, Nexium and Gaviscon and how to successfully use them.

Diagnosing Gastroesophageal Reflux Disease is the first step towards its successful treatment. However, because the symptoms of GERD resemble the ones of other diseases, in many cases people may not suspect that they have it. In recognition of this, the first chapter of the book contains detailed information about the symptoms of GERD and important tips about how to find out whether a person has GERD or not.

This book also contains other important information that is not available anywhere else and that can save a lot of pain and suffering to people with GERD. This includes the role of uncomfortable or hunched posture in allowing acid reflux and the means to avoid it. The effect of constipation on acid reflux is not described in the current literature about GERD and in this book a separate chapter is dedicated on this topic

The book concludes with a chapter that contains strategies for treatment of GERD depending on the type and severity of the symptoms. This chapter can be used as a guide for achieving the best and fastest improvement possible even in the worst cases of GERD.

Chapter 1. The symptoms of GERD

What is GERD?

GERD stands for **G**astro**e**sophageal **R**eflux **D**isease and it is a chronic digestive disorder that leads to a reflux of stomach acid in the esophagus (the food pipe), causing irritation and inflammation. The chronic exposure to stomach acid damages the esophagus or the throat and leads to development of the symptoms associated with GERD. An estimated 10 to 20 million people in the US suffer from GERD. If GERD is not treated it could lead to variety of esophageal problems, including ulcers, bleeding, pain and discomfort in the chest or the back. Chronic acid reflux causes Barrette's esophagus, which is the abnormal growth of intestinal type of cells in the esophagus and can lead to cancer.

The correct diagnosis is the most important first step in successfully treating GERD. Unfortunately, GERD manifest itself in variety of forms and symptoms and it is difficult to diagnose because its symptoms resemble other conditions particularly heart disease or respiratory infections. To make the things even worse from a diagnostic point of view, people may experience only a part of the symptoms at any given time and frequently do not feel heartburn, acid taste, or burning sensations that typically serve as easy giveaways for the presence of the disease.

What are the symptoms of GERD?

GERD causes all kinds of diverse symptoms including persistent cough, a feeling of a lump in the throat, heartburn, chest pain and discomfort, or generally feeling sick and not well. Many of the symptoms of GERD are summarized in the figure below.

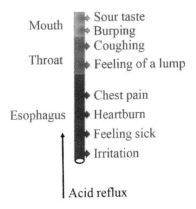

Acid reflux

What symptoms a person experience depends on the intensity of acid damage, the location of the damage (e.g. throat or esophagus, what part of the esophagus etc.) and the frequency and the intensity of the acid reflux. If stomach acid flows up in a region which has not been previously damaged or irritated, the symptoms can be felt as mild irritation. When stomach acid flows on top of acid wounded tissue the result can be sharp pain, spasm or even feeling like passing out.

In the initial stages of GERD people may feel occasionally heartburn, sour taste or burping. Everybody has experience these symptoms one time or another. In healthy people these symptoms appear rarely, for example a few times a year and it is not a big problem, because the reflux of acid is not frequent enough to damage the epithelium of the esophagus or the throat. In contrast, people that suffer from GERD experience acid reflux frequently, ranging from a few times per week, to every day of the week or every hour of the day.

The chronic acid damage that ensues can cause chest pain and discomfort even in the absence of perceptible burning sensation. The acid reflux can make people suddenly feel sick and wasted, without giving any other indications. Because a feeling of burning or acid taste is frequently absent, people may suffer from GERD for years and still may have no idea that they have the disease. A more detailed description of the most common symptoms of GERD are provided below:

Sour Taste

Experiencing sour taste is an indication of acid reflux. However, in most cases of acid reflux sour taste cannot be felt. It is possible that a person gets used to the acidic taste and fails to notice it, or that the acid doesn't go all the way up to the mouth. Because of this the absence of sour taste does not mean that someone doesn't have GERD or acid reflux. On the other hand, feeling acid taste is a good indicator of acid reflux.

Belching and burping

Burping is one of the best indicators of GERD. Of course not everyone that burps have GERD, but burping in combinations with other symptoms (for example chest pain) points towards GERD. Burping occur a few second to a few minutes after the acid reflux itself or after chest pain or other unpleasant symptoms. Burping is the most reliable symptom of GERD that occurs almost always when someone has acid reflux. Not worrisome by itself, burping can be very useful in identification and diagnostic of acid reflux disease.

Irritation of the esophagus

Frequently acid reflux can be felt as a barely perceptible irritation in the chest or the upper abdomen that makes people touch and massage the corresponding area. In many other cases even this feeling for irritation may not be present.

Heartburn

As the name heartburn suggests burning sensation is a one of the most typical symptoms of GERD. Burning sensation can appear suddenly as a result of acid reflux and can be felt in the upper abdomen or more frequently in the chest area. But don't rush to the conclusion that if you don't feel burning you don't have GERD, because frequently acid reflux does not cause heartburn. This is why the absence of burning sensation does not necessary mean that someone does not have GERD.

Chronic cough

Stomach acid refluxed in the throat can damage its lining and cause irritation and inflammation. Coughing usually occurs in the morning after sleeping or after eating. In most cases, the stomach acid can rise up as high as the throat only when people are lying down or sleeping. Because acid reflux occurs during the sleep, people may not be aware of other symptoms of GERD such as burping or heartburn. This is why people may think that they have the flu or another respiratory infection and may not suspect that their cough is caused by acid reflux. If not treated the coughing will persist for months or years. The best way to find out if the cough is caused by GERD is by taking antacids such as Prilosec or Nexium. These drugs alleviate coughing caused by GERD within a week or two after taking.

Feeling of a lump in the throat

If the stomach acid has burned the epithelium below the larynx, the results may not be coughing but a feeling of a lump in the throat even though there is no lump present when the throat is examined. The feeling of a lump is most intense in the morning after sleeping and may gradually decrease during the day. Coughing may be present or not. Other symptoms related to GERD such as heartburn may not be present and in most cases people wouldn't know that this problem is caused by GERD. Taking antacids such as Prilosec or Nexium can lead to an improvement of this symptom.

Chest pain

The reflux of gastric acid can cause damage and inflammation of the esophagus as well. The wounded and inflamed part of the esophagus is frequently located in close proximity to nerves innervating the chest area and the heart. Activating and irritating these nerves during acid reflux is what causes chest discomfort and pain. This can be felt either as chest discomfort throughout the day or as a sudden sharp stabbing pain in the in the middle or the left side of the chest that last for a few seconds. The symptoms are almost indistinguishable of those preceding a heart attack. This is why people experiencing these symptoms should visit the emergency room and later a cardiologist to exclude the possibility of a heart disease. An indication that the chest pain may be caused by GERD is if other symptoms are present, for example burping, heartburn or sour taste. Burping is frequently the only symptom that accompanies chest pain caused by GERD. Prilosec and Nexium alleviate the symptoms of chest pain, but have not immediate effect. It is necessary to take the medicine at least for a week or two to allow the esophagus to heal and inflammation to subside. Even then the antacids do not provide complete protection and chest discomfort may occur even during the period of the treatment.

Suddenly feeling sick or like fainting

The sudden rush of gastric acid into the inflamed esophagus can trigger the nearby located spinal nerves. The result can be a sudden feeling of uneasiness and weakness or a feeling like passing out. This also could be associated with burping and irritation in the chest area. It is important to mention that although GERD can make someone feel like fainting it never leads to actual fainting or loss of conscience. If the latter happens it could be a sign of even more serious condition.

Complications of GERD

It is important to diagnose and treat GERD before the development of the full spectrum of severe symptoms that this disease can produce. If left untreated GERD can produce life-threatening complications. Usually this happens when people do not connect the dots to link their symptoms with acid reflux and as result do not take any steps to treat the disease. The complications that GERD causes can be very unexpected and sometimes even hard to believe. Below we provide a description of known GERD complications:

Dehydration and dizziness

If left untreated GERD may progress towards life threatening condition that requires hospitalization. The chronic acid damage to the esophagus may make the intake of food and liquids difficult. The resulting dehydration and exhaustion may result in dizziness and weakness and in inability to work or even to handle everyday activities.

Inability to sleep

When acid reflux is very intense during the night, you may not able to sleep. In time the ensuing insomnia will contribute to weakness and exhaustion.

Difficulty walking

The esophagus comes in close proximity to the spinal cord and the nerves that controls the movements of the legs and arms. The inflammation caused by acid reflux can migrate from the esophagus to the nearby nerves and as a result people may experience pain or extreme weakness in one or both of their legs. Walking even a short distance can become very difficult.

Respiratory problems and pulmonary disease

The damage and inflammation caused by acid reflux can travel to the respiratory system, where it can cause ear, throat and nose disorders, asthma and bronchospasm, chest congestion, lung inflammation, bronchitis and pneumonia.

Esophagitis and esophageal narrowing

The acid reflux can also cause a severe inflammation of the esophagus, a condition known as esophagitis. Extensive acid damage can cause strictures, scarring and narrowing of the esophagus, which can make swallowing of food difficult.

Barrette's esophagus

The long-term exposure to gastric acid turns the esophageal epithelial cells into intestine-like cells. This syndrome, known as Barrette's esophagus is a precancerous condition that can progress to esophageal cancer.

Esophageal cancer

The chronic exposure to gastric acid can lead to development of esophageal cancer with potentially deadly outcome.

The best advice we can give the reader is to avoid these complications of GERD by taking preventive care. Don't let the situation slip out of control, because then even the best doctors may not be able to help you. The exercise program described in Chapter 3 stops the progression of GERD and prevent the development of all of the sinister complications associated with this disease.

How to find out if you have GERD?

There are cases in which people experience heartburn, burning sensations, acidic taste, burping or others, and it is obviously clear that they have GERD. In other cases, the connection between acid reflux and the symptoms of the disease appear to be not as clear or even probable. This section is dedicated especially to these hard cases and symptoms in order to provide the reader with the necessary information to correctly identify GERD. We begin this section by providing a few real examples, where the link between acid reflux and symptoms was not clear at first, but proven to be correct later.

Case1. Mark has a cough. The cough occurs every morning after sleeping, lasts for 10-30 min and then it subsides. The same repeats after every meal during the day. The coughing has continued already 3 months and there is no sign that it will stop. Heartburn, burping, or chest pain are not present. There is no fever. This condition may be caused by GERD. Mark takes Prilosec for a couple of weeks and feels an improvement.

Case2. Tommy experiences chest discomfort from time to time during the day. Once or twice during this day he feels striking or stabbing sharp pain in the chest area that last for a second or two. The pain sometimes is in the middle of the chest and sometimes on the left. Burning sensation is not present, but he feels slight irritation in the middle of his chest and he burps a lot. He visits the emergency room, but they can't find anything wrong with his heart. Tommy takes Prilosec and within a week he starts to feel better.

Case3. Lisa is watching a movie and she is a sitting in an uncomfortable seat. During the movie she suddenly feels sick. She doesn't feel heartburn or chest pain, but feels like fainting. She also feels like burping. She takes Gaviscon that temporally helps by blocking her acid reflux.

In summary, finding out if a person has GERD is not easy. This disease causes variety of symptoms, many of which are difficult to connect at least at first sight with acid reflux (for example coughing, chest pain, or felling of passing out). To make the problem worse from a diagnostic point of view these symptoms do not appear all at once; a person can have chest pain, but not to cough or he/she may cough, but experience no chest discomfort and pain. Heartburn may be present or not.

FAQs about GERD symptoms and diagnosis

How GERD is diagnosed?

There is no known medical test that can diagnose GERD. In cases of chest pain the doctors focus on finding potential heart problems. If no problems are found then they may suggest GERD, but because no medical test for GERD is available this always remains a proposition and not a conclusive diagnosis.

How to find out whether you have GERD or not?

In the absence of medical test for GERD, the best option is to take Prilosec or Nexium for a week or two. If your condition is improving, there is a good chance that you have GERD. All you need to know about Prilosec and Nexium is included in Chapter 5. Once you know that you have GERD, you need to think about long-term solution, which cannot be provided by the antacids. How to eliminate GERD through exercising is described in Chapter 3.

What symptom is most indicative of GERD?

The answer may surprise many but burping is the only consistent symptom of GERD. Burping occur every time during and after acid reflux. All other symptoms including heartburn, chest paint, feeling sick, acid taste, coughing etc. may be present or not. People usually experience only one or two of these symptoms at the time, in addition to burping. For example, if you have chest pain, burping may be an indication that you have acid reflux, but not a heart attack. Similarly, if you suddenly feel sick or like fainting, the presence of burping may be a sigh of acid reflux and not something worse.

Do you always feel heartburn, when you have acid reflux?

No, people may not feel heartburn or burning sensations, even though they may feel chest pain, feel sick or other GERD symptoms at the time.

You have heartburn, does it mean that you have GERD?

Yes, having heartburn or feeling of burning in the chest or the upper abdomen is indicative of acid reflux and GERD. However, the severity and complications of GERD may not always be associated with the feeling of burning. In many cases people may have severe symptoms of GERD (for example chest pain and discomfort) in the absence of burning. Acid reflux and heartburn also can occur in healthy people from time to time. The difference with people that suffer from GERD is that the latter experience acid reflux very frequently and as a result they sustain a substantial amount of acid damage to their throat or esophagus.

How to find out if your chest pain is caused by GERD or a heart problem?

If you have chest pain and discomfort you need to visit the emergency room and then follow appointment with a cardiologist to find out if there is a heart problem. GERD causes very similar symptoms with the ones caused by heart disease, and based only on the symptoms, the two pathologies are very difficult to discern. Once you have rule out a heart problem as an explanation and suspect that your chest pain is caused by GERD, there are several things you can do. First, when you feel chest discomfort again, observe whether you have other symptoms of GERD, in particularly heartburn or burping. A combination of chest pain with burping or chest pain with burning sensations is indicative of GERD. Second, start taking Prilosec or Nexium for 1-2 weeks to see whether this will reduce your chest pain and discomfort. But most importantly think preemptively and stop GERD by performing the exercise program described in Chapter 3. Doing the exercises will eliminate your chest pain and discomfort and with it the need to visit doctors and hospitals.

Can acid reflux suddenly make you feel sick, even though you don't feel heartburn or chest pain?

The answer may surprise many, but this indeed is very common. When people have acid reflux they may suddenly feel sick and exhausted or like passing out, but they may not feel burning sensations, heartburn or chest discomfort. In these cases, it is difficult to tell if this symptom is caused by GERD or by something else. A giveaway for GERD is that this symptom usually goes together with burping. Prilosec and Nexium can lead to an improvement in a week or two, but this symptom can be eliminated only by doing the exercises described in Chapter 3.

How to find out if your cough is caused by GERD?

Chronic cough that last for months or years can be caused by GERD. Coughing can be the only symptom, without any heartburn, burping or other indications of GERD. The best way to find out if coughing is caused by GERD is to take antacids such as Prilosec or Nexium and observe if coughing subsides within a week or two.

Chapter 2. The cause of GERD

Why healthy people don't have acid reflux?

The production of hydrochloric acid in the stomach is necessary for proper digestions of food and for protection against pathogenic microorganisms that are efficiently killed by the high acidity of the gastric juice. The stomach acid is also harmful to the normal cells of the human body. This is why the stomach cells have evolved specialized mechanisms to cope with the hazardous effect of gastric acid. However, parts of the digestive system including the esophagus (the food pipe) and the throat are not protected against the harmful effects of stomach acid. GERD is caused by the reflux of stomach acid into the esophagus or the throat and the resulting acid damage is to blame for the development of all associated with GERD symptoms. But why gastric acid is refluxed into the esophagus in people that suffer from GERD? In healthy people this doesn't happen even if they stand upside down (people can even drink and eat in a such reverse position!). To understand what happens in GERD lets first examine how the reflux of acid is blocked in healthy people (see picture below).

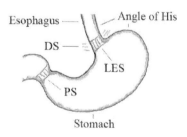

In normal circumstances the reflux of acid is blocked by the lower esophageal sphincter or LES, a special circular muscle that controls the opening of the esophagus into the stomach. In addition, part of the diaphragm wraps around LES and forms an outside sphincter, known as the diaphragmatic sphincter (DS). When the stomach is full the contractions of both LES and DS are necessary to achieve full closure of the food pipe. The exit of the stomach is equipped with another sphincter known as the pyloric sphincter (PS) that controls the movement of the stomach content into the intestine.

The cause of acid reflux and GERD is a malfunction of the lower esophageal and the diaphragmatic sphincters. LES and DS efficiently stop the reflux of gastric acid into the esophagus of healthy people, but in people with GERD these sphincters are leaky. The reason of why LES and DS don't work well in people that suffer from GERD is not well understood.

The stomach has other adaptations to prevent acid reflux. In healthy individuals the esophagus enters the stomach at an acute (sharp) angle, known as the angle of His (see image on previous page). The angle of His traps the food in the stomach and blocks its movement back into the esophagus. The specific shape and the position of the stomach in the abdominal cavity is such that the stomach content doesn't put a pressure on the esophageal entrance and the LES directly. Instead, when the stomach gets full, its expansion leads to a decrease of the angle of His and constriction of the esophageal entrance that facilitates the closure of LES and blocks acid reflux. This is why the prevention of acid reflux require not only the LES, but also the correct position of the stomach in the abdominal cavity, the specific angle of entrance of the esophagus into the stomach e.g. the angle of

His and the relative position of the diaphragm and the diaphragmatic sphincter. This is very important to understand, because altering the position of the stomach or its size and shape renders the LES and the DS ineffective and allows acid reflux.

GERD is caused by a change of the angle of His

The role of the abdominal and diaphragmatic muscles in holding upright posture and GERD

In the normal upright posture as shown below the shoulders are straight, the diaphragm is strong and pushed higher, and the abdomen is straight.

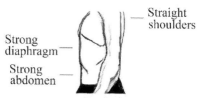

Keeping and holding straight and upright posture throughout the day stops acid reflux and prevents GERD.

Due to a weakness of the diaphragm and the abdominal muscles many people are not able keep a normal straight posture for more than a few minutes resulting in the hunched posture with a loose and bulging abdomen shown below.

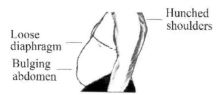

In this posture the shoulders are hunched, the diaphragm is loose and drops down, and the belly is bulging. The deformation of the abdominal cavity leads to repositioning of the stomach, which leads to acid reflux and GERD.

Weakness of the diaphragm and the abdomen alters the angle of His and changes the size and shape of the stomach

The image below depicts changes in the position and the shape of the stomach in people that have a loose diaphragm and abdomen as seen in X-ray pictures and explain how this leads to acid reflux and GERD.

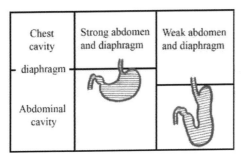

In healthy people with a strong abdomen and a diaphragm the stomach is located in the upper part of the abdominal cavity, where the diaphragmatic sphincter and the lower esophageal sphincter work efficiently together to stop acid reflux. In people with weak abdominal and diaphragmatic muscles, the loose diaphragm moves down and pushes the stomach towards the bottom of the abdominal cavity. To accommodate the internal organs, the belly bulges in front. Also note that the stomach has changed its shape and size. The changes in the position, shape and size of the stomach may result in acid reflux and GERD because of several reasons. First, the angle of esophageal entrance into the stomach (e.g. the angle of His) is altered with the esophagus making a more vertical junction with the stomach and this is conducive for acid reflux. Second, a weak and a loose diaphragm may not support properly the function of the diaphragmatic sphincter. Third, the curvature of the stomach is changed and now the stomach content has to be forcefully pushed upward in order to move into the intestine (see picture). In order to do so the stomach wall and musculature needs to create more pressure. This higher pressure, however pushes some of the stomach content up into the food pipe, causing acid reflux.

Fortunately, these events are reversible. Strengthening the abdomen and the diaphragm straighten the posture, corrects the angle of His and moves the stomach up in its normal position, where it can restore its physiological shape and functions. In Chapter 3 we discuss how to fix the posture by performing exercises to strengthen the diaphragm and the abdominal wall. Performing these exercises is a highly effective way to stop acid reflux and to reverse the symptoms of GERD.

Evidence that GERD is caused by a change of the angle of His

A loose abdominal wall and a prolapsed diaphragm alters the shape of abdominal cavity and misaligns the abdominal organs including the stomach and the esophagus. In the previous section we describe how this altered location alters the angle of His to enable acid reflux, providing an explanation for the development of GERD. What evidence support this explanation?

First, let's consider the fact that the angle of His is anatomically undeveloped in small children. In babies, the esophagus is making almost a vertical junction with the stomach, and as a result, reflux of stomach contents is very common in them.

Second, certain types of surgical procedures (distal gastrectomy) leads to alterations of the angle of His. Patients that have undergone distal gastrectomy are known to develop GERD. It has been reported that that in these patient the angle of His has increased to 109 +/- 22 degrees from 74 +/- 11 degrees, which is the average value in healthy people.

Third, we need to take into account studies that have shown that gaining weight is associated with development of GERD. Overweight people are typically the ones that have loose belly and a weak diaphragm and abdomen and where we can expect that GERD will be especially prevalent, because abdominal weakness is associated with altered angle of His. Indeed, studies have shown that gaining weight increases significantly the chances of GERD and losing weight can reduce the frequencies of heartburn by 40%.

Fourth, acid reflux and heartburn occurs frequently in pregnant women. This happens even if the same women had never had heartburn or other GERD symptoms before, suggesting that altering the location of the abdominal organs may be the cause of GERD.

Fifth, sitting in an uncomfortable seat or holding a hunched posture enables acid reflux. And vice versa taking a good posture prevents acid reflux. This is because a bad posture deforms the natural shape of the abdominal cavity and alters the location, shape and size of the stomach, including the angle of His. The role of posture in GERD is discussed in details in Chapter 4.

Sixth, when people experience heartburn or another symptom of GERD, their abdomen may appear particularly bulging, bloated or swollen. In contrast, when they don't have symptoms of the disease the shape and size of their abdomen is more normal. Have a look in the mirror, when you have acid reflux and see for yourself. Extensive bloating of the stomach may also alter the angle of His.

Seventh, sleeping on the left side blocks acid reflux and sleeping on the right side enables it. This can be only explained if acid reflux depends on the relative position of the stomach in the abdominal cavity and by the effect of the angle of His on acid reflux and GERD.

Eighth, people that have hiatal hernia typically have a severe form of GERD due to altered position of the stomach. In hiatal hernia the stomach protrudes through the diaphragm into the chest area. Most people with hiatal hernia suffer from GERD, because the angle of His is altered and their diaphragmatic sphincter is no longer functional.

Ninth, we have found that exercises that train the abdominal muscles and the diaphragm and that correct the posture and the shape of the abdomen and are also expected to adjust the angle of His eliminate GERD even in its worst form. How to achieve this is discussed in the next Chapter 3.

Chapter 3. Curing GERD through exercising

Currently, GERD is incurable by using conventional medicine. In extreme cases of GERD surgery can be performed that attempts to narrow the esophageal entrance and tighten the lower esophageal sphincter. This is effective against GERD in only 50-70 % of cases. Even, when successful, the symptoms of GERD may come back later within a few months or years. Moreover, the surgery may create other problems such a difficulty in swallowing or vomiting and may lead to chronic stomach bloating. The surgical wounds may get infected and endanger your life. Surgery, is obviously a risky and not reliable option for treating GERD. Pharmaceutical companies have developed drugs that are designed to reduce the damage caused by acid reflux. Antacids medicine such as Prilosec and Nexium block the production of hydrochloric acid in the stomach and may reduce the damage that it causes when it is refluxed into the esophagus. Gaviscon temporarily block acid reflux by creating a foamy barrier. Unfortunately, all antacids that can be bought at the pharmacy are designed to reduce the damage caused by acid reflux and do not treat the underlying causes for the disease. This is why although these drugs can be useful for treating the symptoms of GERD, they do not provide cure for the disease.

GERD can be cured by performing specific exercises

Based on our understanding of the importance of bad posture, abdominal weakness and the angle of His in development of

GERD we have developed specific exercises that strengthens the abdomen and the diaphragm and eliminate acid reflux and all associated symptoms of GERD. Once the posture is corrected acid reflux naturally stops and with it all symptoms of GERD disappear. This can be achieved in about 3-4 weeks of training. Performing these exercises regularly eliminates the need of taking drugs for GERD such as Prilosec, Nexium and Gaviscon.

Not every type of exercising is helpful against GERD. Very dynamic aerobic exercises or certain yoga practices, such as ones that require upside down position of the body may actually facilitates acid reflux and can be harmful for people with GERD.

The exercise strategy to cure GERD is presented in this book for the first time and cannot be found anywhere else yet. By using this strategy, we have obtained great results even in the most severe cases of GERD. This can be demonstrated in the following example, based on real events:

Case 1. George had GERD for many years. He has experienced it all - coughing, chest pain, suddenly feeling not well etc. Many times he had to go to emergency rooms and visits doctors, because he was concerned about his heart. There were periods when he was feeling really sick, when he was not able to work or even getting out of bed was problematic and cases when he was not able to sleep many nights in a row because of acid reflux. After many years of health problems and finally suspecting that he may suffer from GERD, George started taking antacids such as Prilosec and Gaviscon. He started feeling better. However, this didn't cure him. He still had symptoms of GERD at least a few times per week – heartburn, chest pains and discomfort, feeling tired and exhausted, and sometimes he was feeling like passing out. Finding out about the exercises against GERD he started doing them every day. After a month he notice that his figure has improved, that his belly is flattened and that his posture has strengthen. Around this time, he noticed that all the symptoms that he had before were gone, even though he was not taking antacids anymore. He continued exercising and he didn't have any problems for a year even though he had quitted taking antacids. Later, George found a new demanding job and he stopped exercising. After 4 months he started feeling chest pains and heartburn and had to start taking antacids again. He also noticed that his abdomen was weak and bulging again and his posture was hunched. Having no choice, he started exercising again. In a few weeks he was back to normal and healthy with all of his GERD symptoms gone. Ever since George is exercising every day and he doesn't have any symptoms of GERD, even though he is not taking Prilosec and Gaviscon or any other antacids anymore.

Exercises for stopping GERD

People with GERD have very weak abdominal muscles and a feeble diaphragm, and don't have the strength to maintain a correct posture, especially for longer periods of time or throughout the day. The acid reflux occurs as a result of a bad posture and out of place position of the stomach in the abdominal cavity that alters the angle of His (Chapter 2). We have found that a combination of two types of exercises produces the best results against GERD. One set of exercises directly aims at correcting the posture and repositions the stomach, while the second strengthens the abdominal wall.

The latter is necessary to obtain the needed strength to keep and hold a good upright posture throughout the day. We begin with some exercises for correcting the posture, followed by exercises aiming to strengthen the abdominal wall.

Exercises for correcting posture

Exercise 1. Taking a breath followed by contraction of the abdomen wall while standing.

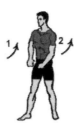

The exercise is performed in two steps: (1) While standing take a deep breath to lift the chest and the diaphragm up. (2) Contract the abdominal wall towards the body and hold until you can. After that exhale and relax the abdomen. Repeat the exercise a few times. Alternatively, you can press with the abdominal muscles a few times before you exhale. Observe your posture in a mirror. While performing the exercise the chest expands and moves up, the abdomen flatten, the shoulders straighten and the stomach moves up and in towards its normal location. The bulging of the belly should be visibly reduced or gone. Performing the exercise leads to unintended straightening of the shoulders. Do not try to intentionally straighten the shoulders. Just using your breathing and abdominal muscles is sufficient to correct the posture. Try to do this exercise in 3-4 series. In every series do the exercise several times for total of 2-3 minutes.

Exercise 2. Breathing followed by contraction of the abdomen wall while sitting.

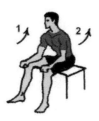

This is similar exercise to the first one but performed in a sitting position. Take a sitting position with hands touching the knees. The body is slightly leaned forward (it works also if you lean the body backwards). The exercise is performed in two steps: (1) Take a deep breath and (2) push your abdominal muscles inwards to the direction of the body. If necessary, you can help your belly by pushing in with one of your hands.

Exercises to strengthen the abdominal wall

Performing the above described exercises to fix the posture can temporally align the abdominal organs and prevent acid reflux. However, maintaining the correct posture during the entire day requires strength of the abdominal muscles that people with GERD lack. This is why it is necessary to perform other exercises that will allow the abdominal muscles to reach the desired strength. Initially, it may be possible to maintain the correct posture for only a few second or minutes, but as you gain more abdominal strength you will find that keeping s good posture for longer periods of time or even for the entire day without a conscientious effort is possible.

Since the problems of GERD primary stems from the loosening of the diaphragm and the upper part of the abdomen (where the stomach is located), the best exercises for GERD are the ones that train the upper abdominal muscles and the diaphragm. The exercise 3 shown below trains the upper abdomen and it is one of the best exercises against GERD.

Exercise 3. Sit ups or crunches with elevated legs (the best exercise against GERD).

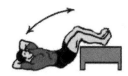

The exercise is performed in two steps: (1) Put your legs piece of furniture (typically a bed or a sofa) as depicted; and (2) with your hands behind the head start doing sit ups. If this is too hard to do, you may keep your arms on the side. If you don't have the strength to do even this, at first you may start with regular sit ups and after gaining some abdominal strength to switch to sit ups with elevated legs. If necessary, use a blanket or a yoga mat for the floor.

Performing sit ups with elevated legs gives excellent results for training the upper abdomen and the diaphragm. Performing 3-4 series for 10 -15 min every day is sufficient to gain substantial strength to the upper abdomen and produces excellent results against GERD. In each series try to do as many sit ups as you can. For most people this number is usually between 10-30. But don't worry if you can do only a few. In a relatively short time you'll be able to do a lot more.

The same exercise can be performed as crunches, instead of complete sit ups. Crunches are half-sit ups. When doing crunches don't move your body all the way to sitting positions but stop in the middle. Crunches train only the abdominal muscles, while the sit ups also pressure the lower back. This is why sit ups sometimes strain the lower back and may cause muscle soreness and pain. We have found that sit ups with elevated legs is very effective against GERD. We suspect that crunches will be also effective, but we have never compared the two. This is why we recommend to start with sit ups with elevated legs. You may try crunches as an alternative and find out which one works best for you. Some people may find exercise 3 to be a difficult one, because they lack the necessary abdominal strength. For them we recommend sit ups or/and crunches in a horizontal position, which are much easier to do (exercise 4-6). These exercises can be performed on a blanket or a yoga mat on the floor. They primarily train the lower abdomen and this is why they are not as good as exercise 3 against GERD that trains the upper abdomen and the diaphragm. However, once people gain the necessary strength they can switch to exercise 3.

Exercise 4-6. Sit ups or crunches in a horizontal position (for people with a weak abdomen)

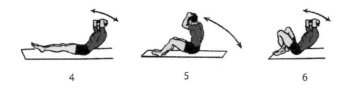

4   5   6

In exercise 4, the legs are straight and they need to be hold by someone or something. Although this is the best known position for sit ups or crunches it is not very comfortable and it also strains the lower back and the legs. For this reason, we don't recommend doing exercise 4. Much better and easier to do are exercises 5 and 6. In exercise 5, the legs are bended at the knees as depicted and exercise 6 is performed with crossed legs. In both cases there is no need for the legs to be hold in place by someone or something. Both exercises can be performed as either sit ups or crunches. To illustrate this, we have depicted a sit up for exercise 5 and a crunch for exercise 6. Performing sit ups or crunches in a horizontal position is not as effective against GERD, because it trains mostly the lower abdomen. Exercise 3 trains the upper abdomen and the diaphragm and it is preferable against GERD.

Some people have strong abdominal muscles and may find that exercise 3 is too easy to do. For them we recommend sit ups from an incline position; exercises 7-9, depicted below.

Exercise 7-9. Sit ups or crunches from an inclined position (advance training for people with strong abdominal muscles).

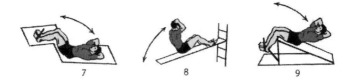

7   8   9

Performing sit ups or crunches in such elevated position can be done by using specially designed benches, which you can find in many gyms. Crunch benches, also known as sit up benches are also available in many sport shops. They are not expensive and can be typically purchased for about 40-100$.

Examples of crunch and sit up benches are depicted below.

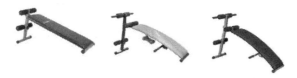

Using crunch benches is a lot more strenuous to the abdominal muscles than exercise 3-6 and may cause temporally unpleasant muscle soreness and lower back pain, especially for people that are just beginning to exercise. This is why we recommend to consider using crunch benches only for more advance training and only after people have already gained substantial abdominal strength.

There are many other exercises that train the abdominal muscles, but currently we haven't tested how beneficial are they against GERD. Many of them can be performed on specialized equipment in a gym (for example exercise 10 and 11 depicted below). These are not absolutely required to do against GERD, but for people that are more enthusiastic about training they can make exercising more entertaining.

Exercise 10-11. Lifting the legs up (exercises for the gym)

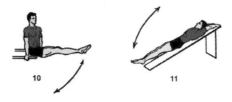

Exercises 10 and 11 are less strenuous on the back and can be performed with no risk for development of muscle soreness or back pain. However, these exercises train the lower abdomen and are not a substitute for training the upper abdomen, which is more effective against GERD (see exercise 3). You may perform these exercises in addition to the ones for the upper part of the abdomen (exercise 3).

Strategy for exercising

For eliminating GERD the best exercises are the ones that train the upper abdominal muscles (exercise 3), in combination with exercises for correcting the posture (exercise 1 or 2). Typical for the sit ups or crunches training the upper abdomen is that the legs are elevated in comparison with the rest of the body. Doing exercises that train the abdomen at home is sufficient to produce excellent results against GERD. But if you' d like to go to a gym, there is no problem because the exercises can be performed in a gym setting as well.

For people that are not enthusiastic about exercising or don't have much time we recommend the following **minimal program** for exercising, that is quite effective against GERD:

Minimal exercise program

Every time do 3-4 series sit ups with elevated legs (exercise 3). In each series do as many sit ups as you can. In between the series perform exercise for correcting the posture (exercise 1 or 2). The whole routine takes only 10-15 minutes. After 3-4 weeks you will observe that many if not all of the GERD symptoms are gone. Exercising more will produce even faster and better results. However, exercising for more than 30 minutes is probably not necessary. We recommend to do the exercises every day if possible, or at minimum 4-5 days a week.

A cornerstone of the exercise program is doing sit ups with elevated legs (exercise 3) that trains the upper abdomen and the diaphragm. However, people that find this exercise difficult and can barely do a few sit ups with elevated legs can temporary substitute it with sit ups in a horizontal position (exercise 5 or 6). After they gain the necessary strength, they can switch to exercise 3.

After training for a while you may find that doing exercise 3 has become too easy. If you can do 50 or more sit ups with elevated legs, we recommend to start doing sit ups or crunches from an inclined position using a sit up (crunch) bench (exercise 9). When using crunch benches be careful not to overdo your exercises, because abdominal muscle soreness or back pain may result. Initially, start with the lowest slope and as you gain more strength you may increase the inclination of the bench.

Advance exercise program

Doing the minimal exercise program is sufficient to eliminate GERD. But there won't be harm done if people do more abdominal exercises and include ones that train the lower or other parts of the abdomen. For example, this may include a blend of exercises 7-11. Don't forget that for GERD the best option is to train the upper abdomen and the diaphragm and that exercises training this part of the abdomen needs to be present. In a gym there may be other machines and equipment that can achieve this. Also don't forget about the exercises for correcting the posture (exercise 1 and 2) that need to be performed in between the series of sit ups or crunches.

Swimming can be helpful for people with GERD

Swimming can be a great way to train the abdominal muscles and the diaphragm and can help people with GERD. Floating and /or swimming on your back is especially useful. This is how it can be done. (1) Take a deep breath and relax with your back on the surface of the water; (2) use the abdominal muscles to straighten your body so that it becomes flat and parallel to surface of the water; (3) periodically take deep breaths and keep floating.

Trying to keep yourself on the surface of the water is all you need to do. In order to achieve this, you need to work with your abdominal muscles to keep the abdomen flat and the body straight and you also need to use the diaphragm when you are taking deep breaths to avoid sinking. This resemble very much exercise 1 for correcting the posture (described above) and it also helps in realigning the abdominal organs and stopping acid reflux.

FAQs about exercising and GERD

Can abdominal exercises cure GERD?

Yes, the described exercises are the best solution for GERD. By stopping acid reflux, the exercises prevent the damage to the esophagus and the throat and eliminate the most severe symptoms of the disease. These include chest pain, suddenly feeling of sickness, chronic cough, heartburn and others.

Does exercising eliminates the need for antacid pills?

Yes, regular exercises for the abdomen and the posture eliminate acid reflux and all associated symptoms of GERD. When this happens taking antacids such as Prilosec, Nexium, or Gaviscon is no longer necessary. Take these drugs only if you have symptoms of GERD.

How does exercising compare with conventional treatment for GERD?

Exercising is vastly superior to taking conventional drugs such as Prilosec, Nexium or Gaviscon. The described exercises treat the cause of GERD; while the above mentioned drugs treat the symptoms of the disease. Taking Prilosec or Nexium decreases the acidity of the stomach content and help reduce some of the damage causes by acid reflux. However, taking these antacids does not prevent acid reflux and cannot eliminate all the damage that it creates. Gaviscon stops acid reflux by creating a foamy barrier over the stomach content. But Gaviscon works only for a limited period of time and as a result allows acid reflux to occur multiple times during the day or the night even if taken regularly. This is why taking Gaviscon, Prilosec or Nexium regularly doesn't eliminate all symptoms of the disease. In the long run taking these antacids is like fighting a losing war, that eventually will be won by GERD. In contrast to this, the presented exercise program eliminates acid reflux 24-hours a day and are the best option for treatment of GERD. In addition to this the long term usage of antacids may produce undesired nutritional and vitamin deficiency, metal poisoning, indigestion, stomach infections or other undesired side effects. In this aspect exercising to prevent GERD is healthy and it doesn't have undesired negative effects and in addition to GERD, it can be beneficial for the heart and the cardiovascular system, the respiratory system and other internal organs and systems.

Does exercising stop the symptoms of GERD immediately?

If you are experiencing heartburn, chest pain or other GERD symptoms doing some crunches won't have much of an effect immediately. This is because it takes time (at least 3-4 weeks) to get sufficient strength of the abdomen to maintain correct posture and to stop acid reflux. Moreover, experiencing chest pain or other severe symptoms of GERD means that there is existing damage to the esophagus. Healing these wounds takes time and it won't happen immediately after exercising. This is why exercising is a long term, but permanent solution for GERD.

How long does it take to feel an improvement?

It takes about-3-4 weeks of exercising. This amount of exercising is required for strengthening of the abdomen and correcting the posture, which in turn stops acid reflux.

How frequently do you need to exercise?

For best results exercise every day. Missing a day or two in a week is not a big deal, but if you want good results exercise as regularly as you can.

How long do you need to exercise?

10-15 minutes per day is the minimum. It is not necessary to do more than 30 min a day.

What is minimal exercise program that works?

You may do 3-4 series of sit ups or crunches with elevated legs (exercise 3). In between the series do exercises for posture (exercise 1).

How to monitor if the exercise program is working?

Observe your posture in a mirror. Is your belly flattened? Are your shoulders straightened? The exercises aim to correct the posture, and they should flatten the belly, move the diaphragm up, and strengthen the shoulders. Regularly observe if exercising produces the desired effects. A more detail description of a good posture is presented in Chapter 2.

If you stop exercising do the symptoms come back?

Yes, GERD may come back. People take actions only when there is a problem. They may have the worst GERD symptoms and eliminate them by doing exercises. Once they don't have the symptoms they are no longer motivated to exercise. In this case GERD may come back within a few months. This is why don't stop exercising, even if you don't have any of the GERD symptoms at the moment.

How to motivate yourself to do the exercises against GERD?

Nothing is more important than your health. So when the time comes forget about everything else and do the exercises. It takes only 10-15 minutes. Anyway, if you don't exercise you are going to spent even more time on visiting emergency rooms, doctors and pharmacies (or think about surgery!). And what is more pleasant, listening to music while exercising at home, or visiting hospitals? If you exercise, you will stop using antacids and save hundreds of dollars every year. It is like you are being paid to exercise. There is no excuse. Just do it.

Chapter 4. Preventing acid reflux by taking and holding a good posture

In this section we discuss how adopting correct posture even for a short while during moments of heartburn or other symptoms of GERD may reduce the severity the symptoms and can help you feel better. Avoiding uncomfortable or hunched positions may prevent acid reflux at a first place. However, doing so is not a substitution for exercising. Exercising is the only way to obtain long term solution against GERD (Chapter 3).

Below we describe how to take and hold a good posture when walking, sitting or sleeping in order to avoid the brunt of acid reflux.

The best posture to take to prevent acid reflux when walking or standing

Try to take the depicted below posture while walking or standing to minimize the chance of acid reflux or when you already have it.

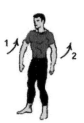

(1) While walking or standing take a deep breath. This moves the chest up, strengthens the shoulders and elongates the abdominal cavity. (2) Then contract the abdominal muscles to flatten the belly. When walking, try to hold more air into

the lungs and keep more tonus on the abdomen. This keeps the body upright and the shoulders straight. Try to walk all the time like this and especially if you are feeling heartburn, chest pain or other symptoms of GERD.

To illustrate this idea let's consider the following situation, inspired by real life experience:

Case 1. James is walking down the street. He suddenly feels not well and is having chest discomfort and pain. He suspects that he just got acid reflux. He notices that he is walking in a hunched posture and his belly feels bloated and loose. He takes a deep breath and pushes with his abdominal muscles. This straighten his entire body and he starts to feel better. This does not eliminate all his symptoms but the situation is now under control and much better than it could have been.

The best posture to take to prevent acid reflux when sitting

Try the depicted below siting position, when you expect to be sitting for a long period of time such as watching a movie or working on your computer.

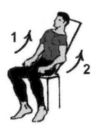

Take a seat and lean your body backwards. (1) Take a deep breath to move the chest up and elongate the abdominal cavity. (2) Push with the abdominal muscles so that the belly flattens. You may also use your hands to help push the abdomen in. Make sure the belly remains flat. Keeping leaned backwards position releases some pressure on the abdomen and keeps the stomach in a position not conductive for acid reflux. Putting your legs up such as on a stool or other furniture can be also helpful, but it is not necessary.

Sitting in a hunched position, where the body is leaned forward is the worst posture that inevitably leads to acid reflux. Even if you keep the torso upright e.g. at a right angle with the legs you still may get acid reflux because this posture creates a lot of pressure on the abdomen. When possible, stand up and walk a bit. The longer you are sitting the higher the chances to get acid reflux.

To illustrate this idea let's consider the following situation, inspired by real life experience:

Case 2. Veronica has noticed that almost every time she goes to the movies she feels sick. This is what happens. While she is quietly watching the movie she suddenly feels an overwhelming rush of weakness and almost feels like fainting. This feeling last a few seconds and then it is gone. This happens a few times during the movie. She also feels like belching. After the end of the movie she feels tired and exhausted and not generally herself. She starts to suspect that her symptoms may be caused by acid reflux and the next time she observes how she is sitting. She leans back on her seat, takes a breath and flattens the abdomen. She finds that by sitting in this position she can go through the entire movie without having acid reflux.

The best posture to take to prevent acid reflux when sleeping

The horizontal position of the body in a bed makes it easier for the stomach acid to reflux into the esophagus. This is why acid reflux occurs more frequently at night while sleeping. Keeping the head elevated such as on double pillow during sleep can help. If you have problems with acid reflux at night sleep only on your left side. Sleeping on the right side is likely to aggravate the symptoms, because it positions the stomach at a location favoring acid reflux. Sleeping in unnatural and uncomfortable positions can significantly worsen GERD. But neither of these measures can entirely stop acid reflux during the night. This can be done only by following the exercise program to train the abdomen and the diaphragm, described in the previous section of the book.

More information about taking and holding a good posture for preventing acid reflux is included in the **FAQs section** below:

FAQs about posture and acid reflux

In what situations do you need to be particularly aware of your posture?

Try to keep and hold a good posture all the time. Unfortunately, that is easier said than done. However, if you don't keep a good posture, you may be getting strong reminders to do so, when you start feeling the heartburn and chest pains of GERD. If you start feeling these symptoms observe your posture. Is your belly loose? Are your shoulders hunched? Correcting the posture when experiencing GERD symptoms can stop acid reflux and make you feel better. The second situation at which you should be particularly aware about your posture is when you expect to be sitting in an uncomfortable chair for a long time, for example if you are going to the movies, sitting in front of a computer or flying on an airplane. Taking and holding a correct sitting position may prevent acid reflux for the entire period of sitting and can save you a lot of pain and discomfort.

Does taking a good posture eliminate GERD symptoms immediately?

Taking and holding a good posture blocks acid reflux and can prevent the appearance of heartburn, chest pain or other GERD symptom. If you already feel these GERD symptoms adopting a good posture may help reduce the discomfort you may experience at the moment and diminish the damage caused by acid reflux, but it is unlikely to eliminate all symptoms of the disease at once. This is because if you are feeling heartburn or chest pain the acid reflux has already irritated and inflamed parts of the esophagus. Time is required to allow the damaged tissue to heal and the symptoms of GERD to disappear.

How effective against GERD is to hold correct posture?

Permanently fixing the posture eliminates GERD and its symptoms. However, this can be achieved only through the exercise program described in Chapter 3. Attempting to keep a good posture even for a short while can be challenging if someone doesn't have enough abdominal strength. It stops acid reflux, when you practice it, but GERD will strike you again when you lose your guard. Nevertheless, attempting to keep correct posture at least for a while can have its uses and be effective in short term prevention of acid reflux. To permanently fix your posture and cure GERD you need to follow the exercise program described in Chapter 3.

Does holding a correct posture for a short while eliminate the need for exercising?

No, exercising is required to obtain long term results and cure GERD. This is because people with GERD don't have abdominal strength to hold permanently a correct posture. They may be successful for a few minutes or hours but eventually they will give up and the acid reflux will take over. Abdominal exercising leads to a permanent fix of the posture. As a result you don't have to think all the time of how to sit or walk and holding the correct posture will come naturally to you.

Chapter 5. Treating GERD with Antacids

Drugs for treatment of GERD and heartburn can be purchased from any pharmacy. Although, GERD cannot be cured by using these drugs, they may provide a short term relieve. Prilosec and Nexium work by blocking the production of hydrochloric acid in the stomach and in such a manner reduce the damage caused by acid reflux. Gaviscon blocks acid reflux by creating a foamy barrier. In this section we discuss how and when to use these drugs in order to achieve the best results.

Prilosec and Nexium

Prilosec and Nexium are antacids that reduce the production of stomach acid. Although, they don't cure GERD, these antacids may reduce the severity of its symptoms. Available over the counter, we recommend to take Prilosec or Nexium especially when experiencing more severe symptoms of GERD such as chest pain or persistent cough.

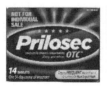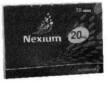

The benefits of Prilosec or Nexium can be illustrated in the following examples, based on real cases:

Case 1. Tony recently doesn't feel very well. He has chest discomfort and a few times during the day he suddenly feels sick and wasted. He is worried that it could be his heart, but he notices that at the moments when he feels sick he starts to burp a lot and he begins to suspect that he has acid reflux. He starts taking Prilosec every day. After a week on Prilosec he definitely feels better. He still burps from time to time and occasionally experience chest discomfort, but he doesn't feel sick or like passing out any longer. He is now more confident that he has GERD, and consider doing exercises against GERD to eliminate all of his symptoms and eventually quit the antacids.

Case 2. Paul is coughing every morning and this has already continued for three months. He has tried all kinds of remedies against respiratory infections, but nothing has helped. He finds out that a chronic cough can be caused by acid reflux. Although he doesn't feel any heartburn he starts taking Prilosec. After a week on Prilosec his cough starts to subside and in a couple of weeks it is almost gone. Paul now knows that he suffers from GERD.

Case 3. Paulina wakes up with very unpleasant symptom. She feels like she has a lump in the throat and she has difficulty swallowing. She starts to worry that she may be getting cancer and goes the doctor's office, but they can't find anything but sour throat. The same feeling is present next morning. She takes Prilosec as suggested by her doctor and she feels like her lump is fast disappearing. Within an hour she doesn't have the feeling of a lump anymore, but she still has a sour throat. Note that the feeling of lump may depend on the continuous presence of acid in the throat and as a result the antacids may work very quickly in resolving this problem. However, they work much slower on reducing chest pain, coughing or other symptoms of GERD, because in these cases there is an injury and irritation in the throat or the esophagus that takes time to subside and heal.

More about Prilosec and Nexium and how to properly use them is discussed in the FAQ section below:

FAQs about Prilosec and Nexium

How Prilosec and Nexium are taken?

Prilosec and Nexium are recommended to be taken in the morning before breakfast. Food intake stimulates the production of stomach acid, so it is important to take the pill before eating. Only one pill per day should be taken. The pill contains slow degradable coating that ensure the continuous release of the active ingredient during the day.

How long can you take Prilosec and Nexium for?

Prilosec and Nexium are not recommended to be taken for more than 14 days in row. After the 14 days you can take a break for 1-2 weeks and continue with taking the medicine afterwards if it is necessary. However, taking these drugs continuously for years may lead to mineral or vitamin deficiency or other detrimental effects on your health.

Does Prilosec or Nexium cure GERD?

No, Prilosec and Nexium don't cure GERD and don't prevent acid reflux. Even with reduced acidity the gastric juice when refluxed can irritate and inflame the esophagus. This is why taking Prilosec or Nexium does not eliminate all the symptoms of GERD. These antacids have only relative effect. For example, in cases of severe form of GERD, taking these drugs will reduce the symptoms only relative to the initial condition. But even if you take these drugs every day you still may get very worrisome symptoms.

You are taking Prilosec every day; does this mean that your GERD problems are solved?

Not at all. Even if you take antacids every day you still may have chest pain and discomfort or to suddenly feel sick or like passing out or not be able to sleep at night, because of acid reflux. This also may have very bad psychological effect, because people may think that they may have heart disease or even die and they still will be visiting emergencies rooms and doctors. Relying only on antacids won't make you healthy. The only way to defeat acid reflux and GERD is by following the exercise program described in Chapter 3 .

When should you take Prilosec or Nexium?

Take Prilosec or Nexium when you experience severe symptoms of GERD such as chest pain, sudden feeling of sickness or persistent cough or in case you have very frequent heartburn. In cases like these taking Prilosec or Nexium may decrease the severity of the symptoms and gives time to the damaged tissues to heal. If you have heartburn only rarely we recommend to use Gaviscon instead (see next section).

How to use Prilosec or Nexium to find out if you have GERD?

GERD symptoms such as chest pain, coughing, suddenly feeling not well etc. can be very difficult to discern from very similar symptoms caused by other diseases. One of the best ways to tell if the symptoms are caused by GERD is to use Prilosec or Nexium. Take 1 pill Prilosec or Nexium every morning before breakfast. If the symptoms are caused by GERD you may observe an improvement in a week or two after starting taking the pills.

Does Prilosec and Nexium alleviate the symptoms of GERD immediately?

No, it usually takes 3-5 days or longer to feel an improvement. The symptoms of GERD are caused by damage and inflammation of the esophagus. After taking the antacids, at least several days are needed to allow the esophageal epithelium to heal.

What is best strategy of taking Prilosec and Nexium?

If the symptoms are very severe such as they have caused you great concern take Prilosec or Nexium for 14 days. If you feel occasional heartburn, discomfort but the symptoms are not very concerning take the medicine for 3-5 days. This usually is enough to get a lasting improvement and you may stop taking the antacids afterwards. If the symptoms reappear, start taking the Prilosec or Nexium again.

If you have GERD should you take antacids all the time?

Prilosec or Nexium should be taken, only if symptoms of GERD are present. Doing the exercises described in Chapter 3 can eliminate the symptoms of GERD and with it the need to take antacids.

Do you need a prescription to buy Prilosec or Nexium?

No, they are over the counter drugs. However, buying them with a prescription may cost less. But if you like to try these antacids, they are easily accessible in any pharmacy without a prescription.

Should you get 20 or 40 mg pills?

Nexium is available as 20 mg or 40 mg pills. We recommend to use the 20 mg pills. The 20 mg pills work well and are almost twice as cheap as the 40 mg pills. The 40 mg pill should be considered only in exceptional circumstances.

What are the side effects of Prilosec or Nexium?

The short term usage of Prilosec and Nexium are not associated with severe side effects. Sometimes they may cause indigestion and abdominal bloating. The prolong usage of antacids may interfere with assimilation of food, minerals and vitamins and increases the chance of gastrointestinal infections.

Are there differences between Prilosec and Nexium?

Prilosec and Nexium contain omeprazole and esomeprazole respectively as active ingredients. They both work equally well, so it doesn't matter which one you chose. The availability of these antacids may differ in different countries. Prilosec is more frequently used in US and Nexium in Europe.

What is the mechanism of Prilosec and Nexium?

Proton pumps are proteins that control the production of hydrochloric acid in the stomach. Prilosec and Nexium inhibit the actions of proton pumps and as such they suppress the amount of acid produced in the stomach.

Gaviscon and Foamy agents

Gaviscon works by creating a foamy barrier that blocks the reflux of gastric acid into the esophagus. The medicine is available as tablets and in liquid form. The tablets need to be chewed to activate the protective foam barrier, while the liquid form of the drug requires contact with gastric acid to trigger the foaming.

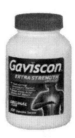

An advantage of Gaviscon over Prilosec or Nexium is that it blocks acid reflux (the antacids do not), but disadvantage is that it has only a short-term effect. Gaviscon need to be taken after eating, because eating or drinking breaks the foam barrier. The advantages of Gaviscon can be illustrated in following examples, based on real events.

Case 1. John is taking Prilosec every day, but this doesn't stop his acid reflux. The situation is especially dire during the night, when every time he tries to sleep is awaken by pain and discomfort in his chest. He feels heartburn and his stomach is bloated and full of gas that drives stomach acid into his esophagus. Sleeping is not possible. This is happening every night and he becomes exhausted from sleep deprivation. He learns about Gaviscon and takes some before going to sleep. This has almost miraculous effect. The gas and acid are no longer driven up into his chest, but are pushed downwards.

He is no longer burping, because the gas now finds its way down. But most importantly, he feels a relief from his chest discomfort and now he can finally fall sleep.

Case 2. Jane has noticed that almost every time during her work meetings, which are held once every week she suddenly feels not very well. She doesn't feel heartburn, but she knows that she has GERD and she is taking Prilosec regularly. She suspects that the symptoms she experiences may be caused by acid reflux triggered either by stress or the uncomfortable sitting position during these meetings. Next time, right before the meeting she takes Gaviscon to prevent her acid reflux. This time she doesn't feel sick during the meeting and now she is certain that her symptoms are caused by GERD.

More about Gaviscon and how to use it is discussed in the FAQ section below.

FAQs about Gaviscon and foamy agents

Does Gaviscon cure GERD?

No, Gaviscon can prevent some acid reflux and heartburn attacks, but it won't cure GERD. It provides only a short term protection. If you have severe symptoms of GERD taking Gaviscon is not going to eliminate them.

I am taking Gaviscon regularly, does this solves all my GERD problems?

Not at all. Taking Gaviscon can help, but you still may have all kinds of worrisome symptoms including chest pain and discomfort, feeling sick and exhausted or others. Taking Gaviscon won't make you healthy. You can defeat GERD only by following the exercise program in Chapter 3.

Does Gaviscon stop acid reflux?

Gaviscon can stop acid reflux by forming an insulating foamy barrier. However, this protection last only 30-40 minutes. It is not possible to take Gaviscon every 30-40 min (it is recommended to be taken no more than 4 times per day). This is why Gaviscon has restricted capacity to protect against acid reflux during the day and provides very limited protection during the night.

When should you take Gaviscon?

Take the foamy agents when you experience heartburn or other symptoms of GERD or preventively when you expect to participate in stressful events or situations. If you have a severe form of the disease take Gaviscon after every meal and before going to sleep.

Does using both Prilosec and Gaviscon produces better results?

Yes, the two drugs complement each other. The former reduces the damage caused by acid reflux, while the latter blocks acid reflux. This is why we recommend to use the combination especially when someone has a severe form of GERD. But using both of these drugs won't make you healthy, because you still will retain a full spectrum of GERD problems. To get rid of acid reflux and GERD follow the exercise program in Chapter 3.

Does Gaviscon alleviate the symptoms of GERD immediately?

Gaviscon can potentially reduce the damage caused by acid reflux. However, if the damage is already done it is unlikely that it will eliminate all the symptoms fast. It may reduce the feeling of burning or heartburn fast, but it won't eliminate chest pain or cough resulting from damage to the esophagus.

How long can you take Gaviscon for?

Taking Gaviscon for years may produce undesired side effects, which are not clearly defined yet. A concern of using Gaviscon is the possibility of aluminum poisoning, specifically if the drug is used for many years.

How to use Gaviscon in case you have a mild form of GERD?

If you have GERD, but have no chest pain or other alarming symptoms, take Gaviscon only after feeling a heartburn. If you plan to participate in meetings, presentations or other events that may increase the stress levels and the chances of acid reflux you may take Gaviscon preventively.

How to use Gaviscon in case of severe form of GERD?

If you have chest pain, persistent cough or other serious symptoms take Gaviscon on regular basis during the day. Acid reflux is more likely to occur after eating and during the night. This is why Gaviscon should be taken after every meal and at bedtime

If you have GERD should you take Gaviscon all the time?

Gaviscon should be taken, only if symptoms of GERD are present. Exercising regularly can eliminate the symptoms of GERD and to obviate the need for Gaviscon.

Tablet vs liquid Gaviscon?

Gaviscon is available as chewable pills and also as a liquid. Both work well for blocking acid reflux. The liquid form doesn't taste very good, but some people think that is more effective than the pills. The pills are easier to carry, so this is an advantage if you are not at home, for example at work or walking outside. Since some people prefer the liquid Gaviscon and some the tablets, we recommend to try both and decide which one works best for you.

How to take Gaviscon pills?

Do not swallow tablets whole. Swallowing the pills does not lead to formation of a foamy barrier and do not provide protection against acid reflux. Instead, chew 2-4 tablets after meals and at bedtime as needed (up to 4 times a day). For best results follow by a half glass of water or other liquid.

How to take the liquid form of Gaviscon?

Take 1-2 tablespoons maximum 4 times a day. Take after meals or at bedtime.

Can you eat or drink after taking Gaviscon?

Eating and drinking after taking Gaviscon is not recommended because it destroys the foamy protective layer and makes the medicine ineffective.

Do you need prescription to buy Gaviscon?

No, Gaviscon is available at any pharmacy without a prescription.

What is the mechanism of Gaviscon?

Gaviscon contains aluminum and magnesium hydroxide. When dissolved these substances form a foamy substance that prevents the reflux of stomach acid into the esophagus. The hydroxides are also bases that work as antacids to neutralize stomach acid.

What are the side effects Gaviscon?

For a short term usage Gaviscon is tolerated well. Indigestion and abdominal bloating are the only problems that have been reported. A concern of using Gaviscon is the possibility of aluminum poisoning, specifically if the drug is taken for many years. Overdosing of aluminum may lead to its deposition in the bones, muscles and brain. Symptoms associated with aluminum poisoning include encephalopathy, speech disorders, tremors or seizures, hypotension, slowed breathing, brittle bones, and others.

Chapter 6. Constipation and GERD

Although constipation is not the cause of GERD, the worst symptoms of GERD may appear during periods of constipation. Constipation increases the frequency and the strength of acid reflux. This is easy to understand if we consider that during constipation the stomach content is not able to move down the digestive tract easily and therefore it is more likely to rise up.

Miralax and GERD

Miralax is an effective laxative that it is widely used against constipation, but the fact that it can help people with GERD has not been described before.

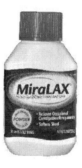

We have found that in cases of severe symptoms of GERD, Miralax can reduce the symptoms of GERD even more so than other heartburn and GERD medicine including Prilosec, Nexium and Gaviscon. Let's consider the following case, based on real life experience:

Case 1. John has frequent heartburn, chest discomfort and pain. He has chest discomfort almost all the time and 5 to 10 times per day he feels a stronger stabbing pain in the chest area. He is taking Prilosec and Gaviscon every day, but the symptoms persist. He is worried that it might be his heart. He goes to the emergency room where and X-ray picture is taken to observe his heart. There is nothing wrong with the heart, but the picture show accumulation of stools in his intestine. This is unexpected for John because he has regular bowel movements. John takes Miralax and this leads to resolution of his constipation in a couple of days. The day after this he starts to feel better, as he no longer feels the stabbing pain and his chest discomfort is reduced. This example illustrates the power of Miralax and the advantage that it can bring over the traditional antacid medicine, especially in cases of constipation.

How to use Miralax and to take advantage of this new treatment option is described in the FAQs section below.

FAQs about Miralax for GERD

Does Miralax cure GERD?

No, Miralax reduced the symptoms of GERD, but it doesn't cure the disease. The only option for curing GERD is by following the exercise program described in Chapter 3.

When to use Miralax for GERD?

Try Miralax for GERD especially if you have more severe symptoms such as chest pain, persistent cough, a sudden feeling of weakness even if there are no obvious signs of constipation. Take Miralax if you suspect that you have constipation irrespective of whether the GERD symptoms are mild or strong.

How effective Miralax is in comparison with Prilosec?

Miralax has a better and a longer effect on GERD in comparison with the antacids. The resolution of constipation allows the stomach content to move into the intestine and this in turn reduces the intensity and frequency of acid reflux. The improvement last for at least a few days to up to a week. During this time, you may feel a big improvement that exceed the effect of the antacids. If you have constipation and take only antacids, you still will experience frequent acid reflux that can cause very uncomfortable symptoms. Miralax reduces the frequencies and intensity of the acid reflux and this in turn could lead to a big relieve from the GERD symptoms.

Does Miralax completely eliminates acid reflux?

No, typically the frequencies of acid reflux may get reduced by 50-80%, but it will not completely disappear. This is why you may have GERD symptoms even if you have taken Miralax.

How long the effect of Miralax last?

After a bowel movement the symptoms of GERD may improve for about a week.

How long after taking Miralax does it take to obtain results against acid reflux?

The result is not immediate and it may take up to a week or even more. Miralax produces a bowel movement 1-3 days after taking. The intensity of the acid reflux usually subsides the day after constipation is resolved, but it may take a few more days or up to a week to feel improvement in other more serious symptoms (for example chest pain and discomfort).

Does acid reflux disappear immediately after constipation is resolved?

People usually don't feel improvement immediately after a bowel movement; in most cases an improvement can be felt next day. This is probably because the stomach content may not move immediately into the intestine. This is controlled by the pyloric sphincter located at the stomach's exit.

Does Miralax works for everybody with GERD?

In case of constipation Miralax is very effective against GERD. If a person does not have constipation taking Miralax may not lead to an improvement. But we recommend to try Miralax just in case, because sometimes it is difficult to know whether someone has constipation or not.

How can you be sure that you don't have constipation?

Constipation sometimes is not very obvious. Even with regular bowel movements every day, a person can be constipated. This occurs when the intake of food exceeds the outtake. We have seen such cases of constipation by X-rays images of the abdomen of patients suffering from GERD. This is why we recommend to try Miralax for GERD even in the presence of regular bowel movements and no obvious signs of constipation.

How Miralax is taken?

Miralax is a powder, that needs to be dissolved before taking. Use the red screw cap of the bottle to measure the amount Miralax to be dissolved. Add the content to half a glass of cool water or other beverage. Drink it and wait 1-3 days for results.

How long does it take to obtain results against constipation?

Miralax produces a bowel movement in 1-3 days.

How frequently should you take Miralax?

After taking Miralax, wait 3 days. If constipation is still present take another dose.

Do you need prescription to buy Miralax?

No, Miralax is available in many pharmacies without a prescription.

Are there natural alternatives to Miralax?

Eating vegetables and fruits is the best way to avoid constipation, because of the fiber they contain. Fiber also is available in tablet form or as chewable pills and candies. Roasted pumpkin is especially good against constipation. Prune juice may also help to resolve constipation. Eating more fiber prevents constipation, but if constipation is already present the best way is to use Miralax.

What are the side effects of Miralax?

It is not known if Miralax have negative side effects when used regularly for years. Miralax in most cases do not have severe short term negative effects. However, people have reported nausea, abdominal cramping, bloating, upset stomach, gas, dizziness and increased sweating after taking Miralax. This is why it is better to control constipation by eating more natural fiber and to use Miralax only when it is necessary.

Chapter 7. Other factors influencing GERD

Food

There is a lot of literature of how to control GERD by following a diet and avoiding specific foods. In case that you experience symptoms of GERD such as frequent heartburn, chest pain or other alarming symptoms you should avoid some types of foods, as described below. Also you should not eat or drink anything if possible at least two hours before going to sleep. With this said, there are many types of food that you can eat if you have GERD and there is no need to restrict your diet to blunt or tasteless food. Moreover, the described in Chapter 3 exercises eliminate GERD and this makes the choice of food less important. If people have symptoms of GERD we recommend that people pay more intention of what they eat. If people don't have symptoms as a result of strengthening of the abdomen and the diaphragm they can eat any food. But even then we recommend to avoid the worse foods for GERD such as very fatty foods or drinking carbonated drinks, which anyway are hazardous for your health.

Foods that need to be avoided at all costs:

Fatty foods such as fatty steaks, fried oily foods, mayonnaise, hamburgers, fries or other fatty fast food can trigger horrifying heartburn attacks. Avoid these foods at any cost. As a general rule avoid any food that shines, because of the fat it contains. In many cases avoiding these fatty foods comes naturally for people that suffer from GERD, because subconsciously they have associated these foods with the acid reflux disease and may feel nauseous only by the look of the fat. Don't invite people suffering from GERD to steak house or fast food restaurants!

Yogurt containing live cultures. Yogurt, generally speaking is a healthy food. However, in people suffering from GERD it may trigger acid reflux and heartburn, especially at night. The metabolic activity of live bacteria in the yogurt is responsible for fermentation processes that may cause bloating of the stomach. The pressurized stomach content may erupt under the pressure into the esophagus and cause acid reflux. For the same reason avoid any probiotic drinks or supplements.

Carbonated drinks. Coke or other soda drinks cause stomach bloating. The pressure build in the stomach by the gas dissolved in the carbonated drinks leads to terrible acid reflux. Avoid these drinks at all costs.

Foods that are well tolerated, but you need to be somewhat careful with:

Spicy food. Contrary to the popular belief, spicy foods are well tolerated by people that suffer from GERD. We recommend to avoid extremely spicy or hot foods, for example such as served in some Mexicans or Indian restaurants. With this said the food need not be blunt and tasteless. Don't give up on tasty food because of GERD!

Fruit Juices. Drinking one or two cups of fruit juice doesn't provoke acid reflux. However, drinking larger amounts of juice such as 1-2 litters at once could create problems. The fermentation of sugar or high fructose glucose syrup that is present in the juice, leads to production of gas, abdominal bloating and ultimately acid reflux. People with GERD should preferably drink water, but 1 -2 cups of juice from time to time is not a problem. Avoid drinking a lot of juice especially before going to sleep.

Bread and other grain products. Eating bread and other bakery product in the short run is good for people with GERD. These foods absorb a lot of stomach fluid making more difficult for the stomach acid to reflux into the esophagus. In the longer run, the grain foods may cause fermentation and abdominal bloating. For that reason, avoid consuming large amounts of grain foods at once, but smaller amounts can be well received.

Fish and chicken. Fish and chicken are well tolerated, and they do not have obvious positive or negative effects on GERD. They are excellent substitutes for pork and beef, which are not particularly good for people with GERD.

Dairy products. Dairy products like cheese are well tolerated and don't create problems with people with GERD. However, avoid consuming yogurt containing live cultures, because it may lead to stomach bloating and strong acid reflux. If you have lactose intolerance do not consume milk and any other dairy products, because the gas and bloating that these foods produce facilitate acid reflux.

Foods that are good for people with GERD:
Ice cream. Having ice cream can temporally relieve heartburn, possibly by cooling down the stomach. Ice cream is as good as Gaviscon. Ice cream, of course, is much tastier alternative to Gaviscon.

Cold water. Drinking half a cup of cold water relives heartburn, but it is not as effective as ice cream. The improvement last only a few minutes.

Vegetables and Fruits. Vegetables and fruits are good for people with GERD or at least are well tolerated. One of the reasons for this is that they are rich in fiber. The fiber creates a mesh in the stomach, which is more difficult to regurgitate back into the esophagus. Consuming lettuce (the best is without seasoning, because it may trigger acid reflux) is very good. Cabbage in moderated amounts is good, but when consumed in large quantities is negative. Other vegetables and fruits can be consumed without obvious positive or negative effects. These include cucumbers, carrots, tomatoes, apples, peaches. Pears are good because of their natural alkaline composition. Some people may get gassy and bloated after consuming large amount of fruits and vegetables and this may add up to their acid reflux problems.

Stomach bloating

Stomach bloating is a major factor that contribute to GERD. Bloating is caused by production of gas in the digestive system, and it is a result of metabolic activity of microorganisms that reside in the digestive tract. The production of too much gas in the stomach may lead to formation of a combustible mixture of gas and gastric acid that is ready to erupt into the esophagus under the pressure. Part of the gas is released by burping, and this is why burping is one the best diagnostic indicators of GERD. The production of gas may depend on the species of microorganisms that inhabit the digestive tract, but there is no conclusive evidence that the presence of specific species may be linked to GERD. Some have suggested that *Helicobacter pilori* is the cause of GERD, but it remains to be determined if this is the truth. Alteration of the digestive microflora by taking probiotics in theory may sounds as a good idea, but in practice haven't produced any good results at least in our hands. On the contrary, taking probiotics have always led to severe worsening of acid reflux disease, probably because the intake of billions of microorganism at once leads to production of a lot of gas and abdominal bloating. Preventing bloating can be very helpful in fighting GERD and there are a few tricks that can be used. First try not to overeat. Eating smaller portions, but more frequently reduces bloating and frequencies of acid reflux. Second do not drink any carbonated drinks, because they introduce a lot of gas and cause significant bloating. Third, do not eat yogurt that contains live bacteria. The yogurt contains billions of bacteria and when digested at once they may cause fermentations and production of a lot of gas and abdominal bloating. Consuming diary product such as cheese and milk can worsen GERD in case of lactose intolerance.

Uncomfortable sitting position

Sitting for a long time in a hunched or an uncomfortable position creates a lot of problems if you have GERD. For example, going to the movies and sitting for a couple of hours in an uncomfortable seat may lead to terrible acid reflux. The same thing can happen if you are sitting for hours in front of a desk or a computer at the office. The reason behind this is that the unnatural sitting position deforms the shape of the abdominal cavity and allows repositioning of the stomach in a location permissive of acid reflux. How to avoid this problem? First try not seat for a very long time in one place. If you are at the office don't seat for hours at one place, but regularly stand up and walk a bit. When sitting observe the best posture for preventing acid reflux (Chapter 4.) And of course use a conformable chair. However, the only way to permanently solve this problem is by performing exercises against GERD (Chapter 3).

Stress

Stress is not the cause of GERD. However, stress can worsen the symptoms of GERD and increases the chances of acid reflux. Acid reflux is more likely to happen during stressful events such as public speaking, presentations, meetings etc. In cases like this consider taking Gaviscon preventively. Drinking a bit of water if you are experiencing acid reflux can also bring a temporal relief. Coping and reducing the stress is important in dealing with GERD. Physical activities and sports are a great way to melt the stress and to experience less acid reflux. The teaching of eastern philosophy such as Zen is a great way of dealing with the stress.

Chapter 8. Treatment strategy for GERD

What to do when you feel heartburn or another symptom of GERD?

If you feel heartburn, chest discomfort or other symptoms that may be caused by GERD, first have a look at the shape and size of your abdomen. Observe if the abdomen is loose and bloated, and whether the diaphragm is relaxed and out of tonus. If this is the case try to correct your posture by taking a deep breath and contracting the abdominal wall to flatten the belly, as previously described in Chapter 4. If you are sitting in an uncomfortable seat lean back, take a deep breath and flatten the abdomen. If necessary, use your hands to push on the abdomen down to mold its normal size and shape. Most importantly consider doing the exercises against GERD described in Chapter 3. The exercises may not have immediate effect, but in a period of 3-4 weeks, they will stop your acid reflux and associated with it symptoms. In severe cases of GERD, in addition to the above mentioned techniques, we recommend the usage of the conventional antacid drugs such as Prilosec and Gaviscon (Chapter 5). They help reduce the damage caused by acid reflux and could make you feel better in the short run. In addition, using laxatives, such as Miralax is helpful in cases where acid reflux is very strong due to a constipation. By following the exercise program described in Chapter 3 you can get rid of acid reflux and GERD. After this is accomplished you will be able to stop taking antacids. The treatment strategy may depend on severity of GERD and the types of symptoms that someone experience. Below we discuss the best strategies for treatment applied to specific cases of GERD.

Treatment strategies depending on the type and severity of GERD symptoms

Case 1. A severe form of GERD with chest pain and discomfort

When a severe form of GERD is present using conventional treatments in addition to exercising is the best option. In this form of GERD, acid reflux occurs many times during the day and the night. There is chest discomfort and from time to time a sharp pain in the chest area, that can be felt for a second or two, more frequently on the left side, but sometimes in the middle side of the chest as well. If not treated the symptoms can become even worse. You may not be able sleep at night because of acid reflux, you may not able to eat and even drink well, you will become exhausted and sick, dehydrated and dizzy. Even doing the everyday chores may become very difficult. What should you do? The first step is to find out if you have GERD or not. For that purpose, start taking Prilosec or Nexium (1 pill before breakfast) for at least 14 days (Chapter 5). These drugs are effective in reducing the symptoms of GERD and you may feel an improvement within a week or two. Starting to feel better is a good indication that the symptoms you have are caused by acid reflux. Second, start taking Gaviscon after every meal and before going to sleep (Chapter 5). The foamy agents can provide additional protection against acid reflux. Third, take Miralax, because constipation leads to particularly strong and frequent acid reflux and may be involved especially in the severe forms of GERD (Chapter 6). Fourth, taking all these drugs may help you feel better in the short run, but won't cure your GERD. This is why you should consider starting the exercises against GERD described in Chapter 3. Strengthening the abdomen and improving the posture stops acid reflux and in time will eliminate the symptoms of GERD. Be patient. When you have symptoms continue taking the antacids, but when the symptoms disappear stop the drugs, but continue exercising.

Case 2. A severe form of GERD that makes you feel very sick

In some cases, the acid reflux is not felt as a chest pain or heartburn. Instead, you suddenly may feel weakness or feel like fainting. It lasts from a few seconds to a few minutes, but afterwards you may feel tired and not very well. In cases like this we recommend the same strategy as in case 1, which include combination of exercising and conventional treatment options.

Case 3. GERD with chronic cough

By damaging the epithelium of the throat the acid reflux may cause coughing that if left untreated will continue for many months or years. If you have chronic cough, we recommend to start with Prilosec or Nexium (Chapter 5). Take these antacids for 14 days and observe if you feel an improvement. This is the best way to find out if the cough is caused by GERD. If this turns out to be the case start doing the exercises against GERD described in Chapter 3. In time you will find that you can stop the antacids and your cough will not comeback.

Case 4. GERD with frequent heartburn

If you are experiencing burning sensation frequently (at least a few times per week), but you don't have chest pain or other alarming symptoms, we recommend to take Prilosec or Nexium for 3-5 days (Chapter 5). If symptoms are gone after that stop taking the antacids. But if symptoms are present continue taking the drugs. Take Gaviscon only when you feel heartburn. Most importantly, start doing the exercises to prevent acid reflux described in Chapter 3. When the symptoms disappear you will be able to stop taking any drugs against GERD.

Case 5. **GERD with infrequent heartburn**

If you have heartburn only rarely (for example once per week or once per month) it is not necessary to take Prilosec or Nexium. You may take Gaviscon, but only when you experience a heartburn (Chapter 5). Most importantly continue exercising against GERD, because this will keep the disease in check (Chapter 3). Observe your posture, especially when you are sitting in an uncomfortable seat such as in a movie theater or in an airplane (Chapter 4).

Case 6. **You had GERD, but recently you don't have any symptoms**

In the past you had very severe form of GERD, but now all of the symptoms are gone. In this case don't take any drugs, but continue exercising as described in Chapter 3, because otherwise the symptoms may comeback.

Comments & feedback

If this book was helpful to you, please tell your friends about the angle of His and leave a review on Amazon. This can inform and help other people with GERD

Thank you and good luck!

Printed in Great Britain
by Amazon

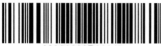